Fresh and Fit Cookbook for Everyday Health

A Guide to Nutritious and Delicious Meals

BY

Alex Aton

Licensing Information

Table of Contents

Introduction.. 5

1. Grilled Chicken with Lemon Basil Pasta 8

2. Roasted Salmon with Brussels sprouts and Sweet Potatoes
....10

3. Quinoa and Black Bean Salad 12

4. Greek Salad with Grilled Chicken 14

5. Chicken and Vegetable Stir Fry..................................17

6. Baked Sweet Potato with Black Beans and Avocado 20

7. Turkey and Vegetable Chili 23

8. Shrimp and Broccoli Stir Fry 26

9. Mediterranean Chicken and Vegetable Skewers 28

10. Spicy Peanut Tofu and Vegetable Stir Fry......................30

11. Lentil Soup with Spinach and Tomatoes........................33

12. Baked Cod with Tomatoes and Olives...........................36

13. Quinoa Fried Rice with Vegetables and Shrimp 38

14. Chicken and Broccoli Alfredo...................................41

15. Greek Yogurt Chicken Salad......................................44

16. Baked Lemon Herb Chicken with Roasted Vegetables ...46

17. Sweet Potato and Black Bean Enchilada........................49

18. Creamy Tomato Soup with Grilled Cheese Croutons......52

19. Grilled Shrimp Taco with Avocado Salsa.......................55

20. Broiled Salmon with Asparagus and Lemon Butter 58

21. Zucchini Noodles with Pesto and Shrimp.......................61

22. Slow Cooker Chicken and Vegetable Soup.....................63

23. Roasted Butternut Squash and Brussels Sprout Salad 65

24. Easy Quinoa and Vegetable Stuffed Pepper....................68

25. Vegan Lentil Soup 71

26. Spinach and Feta Stuffed Chicken Breast.......................74

27. Roasted Vegetable and Quinoa Salad.............................77

28. Greek Chicken Bowl with Roasted Vegetables and Lemon Tahini Sauce...80

29. One-Pan Balsamic Chicken with Roasted Vegetables.....83

30. Cauliflower Fried Rice with Vegetables and Shrimp 86

My Words 89

Introduction

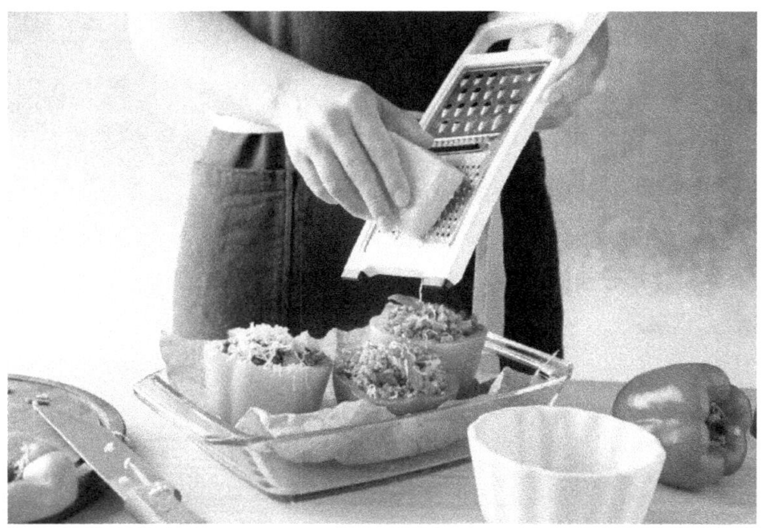

Welcome to Healthy Eating Made Easy! Are you tired of feeling overwhelmed when it comes to meal planning and healthy eating? Look no further! This cookbook is packed with nutritious and delicious recipes that will make healthy eating a breeze. Whether you are a seasoned cook or a beginner in the kitchen, these recipes are easy to follow and will leave you feeling satisfied and energized. With a month's worth of complete menus, you will never have to wonder what to make for dinner again. From savory breakfasts to hearty dinners and even sweet treats, the cookbook has something for everyone. So, grab your apron and let us get cooking!

30 Famous Recipes of Healthy Food that Are Easy to Cook:

1. Grilled Chicken with Lemon Basil Pasta
2. Roasted Salmon with Brussels sprouts and Sweet Potatoes
3. Quinoa and Black Bean Salad
4. Greek Salad with Grilled Chicken
5. Chicken and Vegetable Stir Fry
6. Baked Sweet Potato with Black Beans and Avocado
7. Turkey and Vegetable Chili
8. Shrimp and Broccoli Stir Fry
9. Mediterranean Chicken and Vegetable Skewers
10. Spicy Peanut Tofu and Vegetable Stir Fry
11. Lentil Soup with Spinach and Tomatoes
12. Baked Cod with Tomatoes and Olives
13. Quinoa Fried Rice with Vegetables and Shrimp
14. Chicken and Broccoli Alfredo
15. Greek Yogurt Chicken Salad
16. Baked Lemon Herb Chicken with Roasted Vegetables
17. Sweet Potato and Black Bean Enchilada
18. Creamy Tomato Soup with Grilled Cheese Croutons
19. Grilled Shrimp Taco with Avocado Salsa
20. Broiled Salmon with Asparagus and Lemon Butter
21. Zucchini Noodles with Pesto and Shrimp
22. Slow Cooker Chicken and Vegetable Soup
23. Roasted Butternut Squash and Brussels sprouts Salad
24. Easy Quinoa and Vegetable Stuffed Bell Pepper

25. Vegan Lentil Soup

26. Spinach and Feta Stuffed Chicken Breast

27. Roasted Vegetable and Quinoa Salad

28. Greek Chicken Bowl with Roasted Vegetables and Lemon Tahini Sauce

29. One-Pan Balsamic Chicken with Roasted Vegetables

30. Cauliflower Fried Rice with Vegetables and Shrimp

1. Grilled Chicken with Lemon Basil Pasta

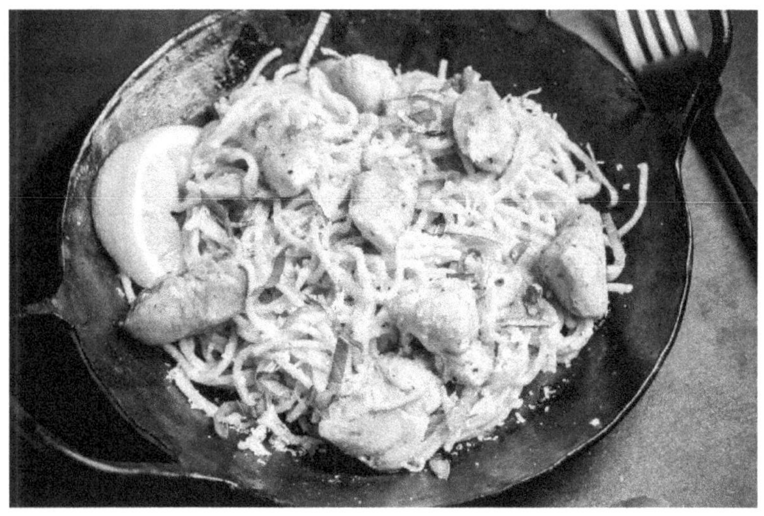

Grilled Chicken with Lemon Basil Pasta is the perfect combination of succulent grilled chicken and fragrant zesty pasta. The chicken is marinated to perfection, while the pasta is cooked al dente and tossed with basil and lemon zest. The result is a dish bursting with flavor and texture that will leave you feeling satisfied and craving more.

Prep Time / Cooking Time: 55 Minutes

Serving Size: 2 Persons

Ingredient List

- 1 boneless are skinless chicken breast
- 1/2 cup uncooked pasta
- 1/4 cup chopped fresh basil leaves
- 1/4 cup lemon juice
- 2 tablespoons olive oil
- 1 minced garlic clove
- Salt and pepper to taste

XXXXXXXXXXXXXXXXX

Instructions

a) Preheat a grill to medium to high heat.

b) Season the chicken breast to taste.

c) Grill the chicken for 6-8 minutes on each side or until cooked through.

d) While the chicken is grilling, cook the pasta according to the package instructions.

e) Once the pasta is cooked, drain and set it aside.

f) In a mixing bowl, whisk together the lemon juice, olive oil, garlic and basil.

g) Add the pasta to the mixing bowl and mix it with the dressing.

h) Serve the chicken with the lemon basil pasta.

2. Roasted Salmon with Brussels sprouts and Sweet Potatoes

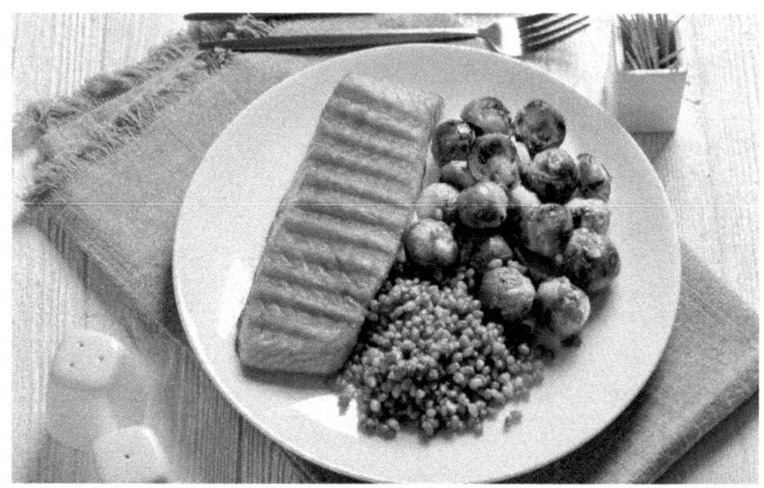

Roasted Salmon with Brussels sprouts and Sweet Potatoes is a healthy and delicious dish that is easy to prepare. The salmon is seasoned with herbs and spices and then roasted to perfection alongside Brussels sprouts and sweet potatoes. The dish is packed with nutrients, including omega-3 fatty acids from the salmon and vitamins A and C from the vegetables. It is a satisfying and flavorful dinner option that is perfect for a cozy night in or a family meal.

Prep Time / Cooking Time: 55 Minutes

Serving Size: 2 Persons

Ingredient List

- 1 salmon fillet
- 4 Brussels sprouts
- 1 small sweet potato
- 1 tablespoon olive oil
- Salt and pepper to taste

XXXXXXXXXXXXXXXXX

Instructions

a) Preheat the oven to 400°F (200°C).

b) Put a baking sheet with aluminum foil.

c) Cut the Brussels sprouts in half and slice the sweet potato into small cubes.

d) Place the vegetables on the baking sheet. Drizzle with the olive oil and season to taste.

e) Mix well. Then, spread the vegetables out in a single layer.

f) Place the salmon on top of the vegetables. Season to taste.

g) Roast for 25-30 minutes or until the salmon is cooked through and the vegetables are tender.

h) Serve hot.

3. Quinoa and Black Bean Salad

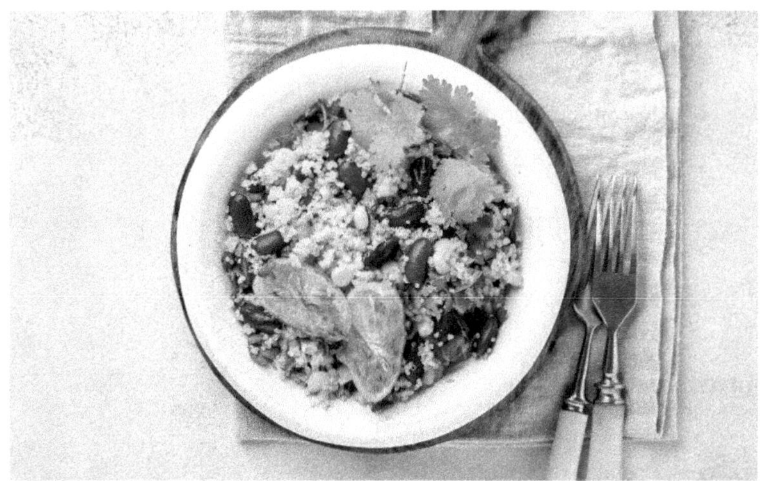

Quinoa and Black Bean Salad is a nutritious and flavorful dish that is perfect for a healthy lunch or dinner. The salad is made with quinoa, vegetables and a tangy dressing made with lime juice. It is a great source of plant-based protein, fiber and vitamins, making it a satisfying and healthy meal option. The dish is easy to prepare and can be customized with your favorite toppings and add-ins.

Prep Time / Cooking Time: 55 Minutes

Serving Size: 2 Persons

Ingredient List

- 1/6 cup quinoa
- 1/6 cup canned black beans
- 1/4 cup cherry tomatoes
- 1/6 cup red onion
- 1 tablespoon lime juice
- 1 tablespoon olive oil
- 1/4 cup diced red bell pepper
- 1/4 cup chopped fresh cilantro
- Salt and pepper to taste

XXXXXXXXXXXXXXXXX

Instructions

a) Cook the quinoa according to the package instructions and set it aside to cool.
b) In a mixing bowl, combine the black beans, quinoa, red onion, cherry tomatoes, red bell pepper and cilantro.
c) In a separate small bowl, put the lime juice, olive oil and salt and pepper to make the dressing.
d) Pour the dressing over the salad. Then, combine well.
e) Serve and enjoy!

4. Greek Salad with Grilled Chicken

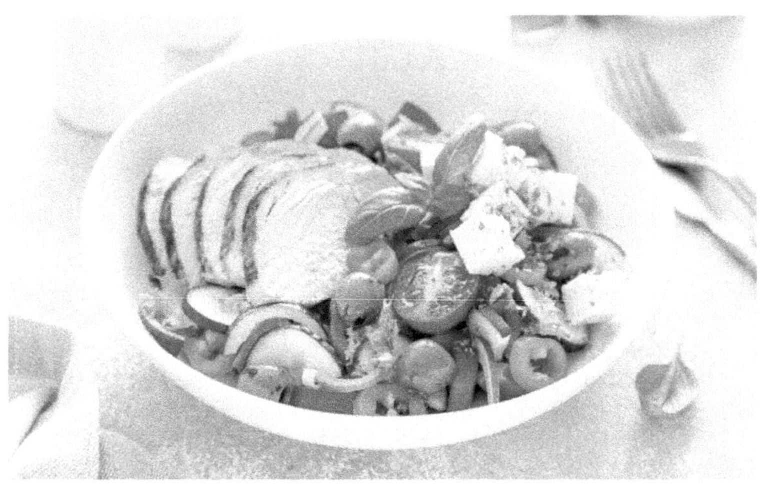

Greek Salad with Grilled Chicken is a fresh and flavorful dish that is perfect for a light and healthy meal. The salad is made with romaine lettuce, cherry tomatoes, cucumber, kalamata olives and feta cheese, topped with grilled chicken. It is packed with protein, vitamins and fats, making it a satisfying and nutritious option. The dish is easy to prepare and can be enjoyed as a lunch or dinner or even as a side dish for a barbecue or picnic.

Prep Time / Cooking Time: 55 Minutes

Serving Size: 2 Persons

Ingredient List

- 2 chicken breasts
- 1 teaspoon dried basil
- 1 teaspoon dried oregano
- 1 teaspoon garlic powder
- 1/2 teaspoon salt
- 1/4 teaspoon black pepper
- 2 tablespoons olive oil
- 4 cups chopped romaine lettuce
- 1 cup halved cherry tomatoes
- 1/2 sliced red onion
- 1/2 cup sliced cucumber
- 1/2 cup sliced kalamata olives
- 1/2 cup crumbled feta cheese

XXXXXXXXXXXXXXXXX

Instructions

a) Preheat a grill pan over medium-high heat.

b) In a mixing bowl, combine the oregano, basil, garlic powder, salt, black pepper and olive oil. Mix well.

c) Add the chicken breasts to the mixing bowl and coat them well with the mixture.

d) Grill for 6-8 minutes per side or until cooked through.

e) Let the chicken rest for 5 minutes before slicing it into strips.

f) In a salad bowl, combine the romaine lettuce, cherry tomatoes, red onion, cucumber, kalamata olives and feta cheese.

g) Add the chicken and toss well.

h) Serve and enjoy!

5. Chicken and Vegetable Stir Fry

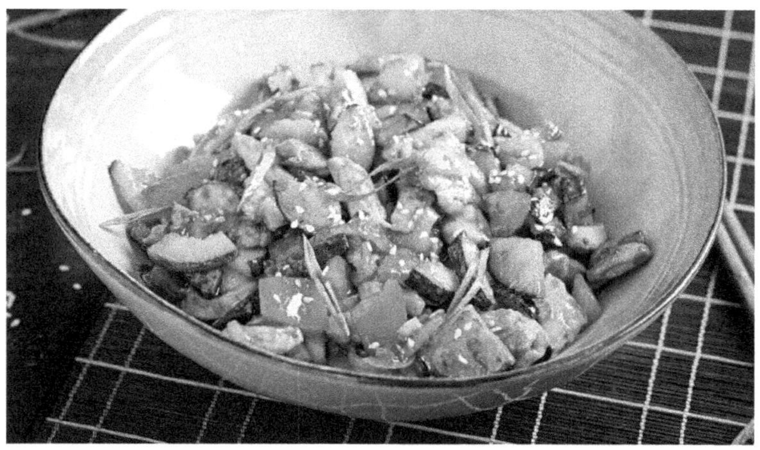

Chicken and Vegetable Stir Fry is a quick and easy dish that is perfect for busy weeknights. It is made by stir-frying tender chicken and fresh vegetables, such as broccoli, bell pepper and onion, in a flavorful sauce made with soy sauce, garlic and ginger. The dish is a great source of protein and nutrients and can be served over rice or noodles for a satisfying and delicious meal.

Prep Time / Cooking Time: 55 Minutes

Serving Size: 2 Persons

Ingredient List

- 2 sliced boneless and skinless chicken breasts
- 1 sliced red bell pepper
- 1 sliced yellow bell pepper
- 1 sliced onion
- 2 cups broccoli florets
- 1/4 cup soy sauce
- 2 tablespoons honey
- 2 tablespoons rice vinegar
- 1 tablespoon cornstarch
- 1 tablespoon vegetable oil
- 1 teaspoon minced garlic
- 1 teaspoon minced ginger
- Salt and pepper to taste

XXXXXXXXXXXXXXXXX

Instructions

a) In a small bowl, whisk together the honey, rice vinegar, soy sauce, cornstarch and 1/4 cup of water. Set aside.

b) Heat the vegetable oil in a wok over medium-high heat. Add the chicken breasts and cook them until browned, about 5-7 minutes. Remove from the wok and set aside.

c) Add the garlic and ginger, then cook for 1-2 minutes or until fragrant. Add the bell peppers, onion and broccoli. Stir-fry for 5-7 minutes or until the vegetables are tender.

d) Add the chicken back to the wok and pour in the mixture. Stir-fry for an additional 2-3 minutes or until the sauce has thickened and the chicken is cooked through.

e) Season with to taste.

f) Serve hot.

6. Baked Sweet Potato with Black Beans and Avocado

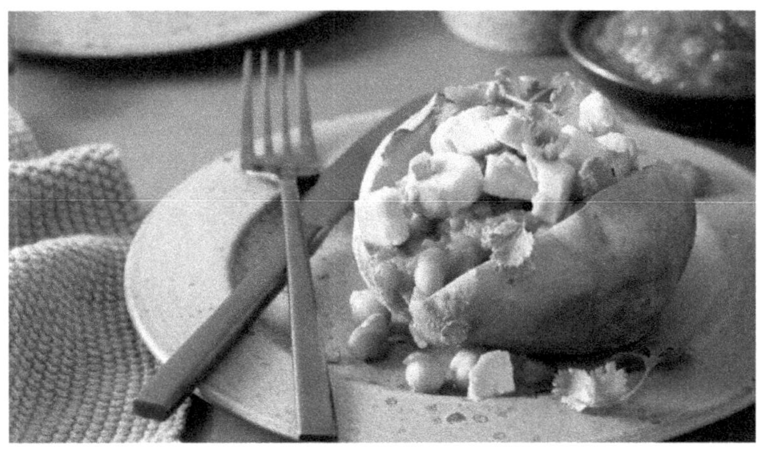

Baked Sweet Potato with Black Beans and Avocado is a healthy and delicious dish that is perfect for a meatless dinner option. It is made by baking sweet potato until tender, then topping it with black beans and avocado. It is a great source of fiber, protein and fats, making it a satisfying and nutritious meal. The dish is easy to prepare and can be customized with your favorite toppings and add-ins.

Prep Time / Cooking Time: 55 Minutes

Serving Size: 2 Persons

Ingredient List

- 2 medium sweet potatoes
- 15 ounces drained and rinsed black beans
- 1 diced avocado
- 1/4 cup chopped cilantro
- 1/4 cup diced red onion
- 1/4 teaspoon cumin
- 1/4 teaspoon chili powder
- 1/4 teaspoon garlic powder
- 1 tablespoon olive oil
- Salt and pepper to taste

XXXXXXXXXXXXXXXXX

Instructions

a) Preheat the oven to 400°F.

b) Wash the sweet potatoes and pierce them several times with a fork.

c) Wrap each sweet potato in aluminum foil. Then, place on a baking sheet.

d) Bake the sweet potatoes for 45-50 minutes or until they are soft and cooked through.

e) While baking, prepare the topping. In a mixing bowl, combine the black beans, avocado, cilantro, red onion, cumin, chili powder, garlic powder, olive oil and salt and pepper. Mix well.

f) Once the sweet potatoes are cooked, remove them from the oven and let them cool for a few minutes.

g) Slice the sweet potatoes in half lengthwise and use a fork to mash the flesh slightly.

h) Top each sweet potato half with the topping.

i) Serve immediately and enjoy!

7. Turkey and Vegetable Chili

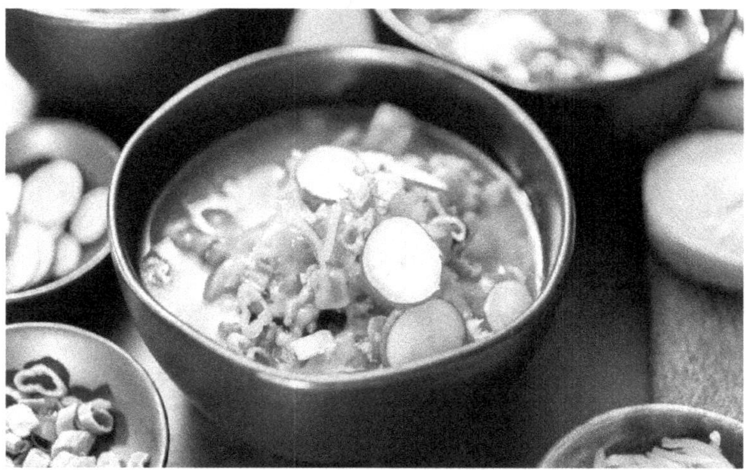

Turkey and Vegetable Chili is a hearty and healthy dish that is perfect for a cozy night in. The chili is made with turkey, vegetables and a blend of spices, then simmered until the flavors meld together. It is a great source of protein, fiber and vitamins, making it a satisfying and nutritious option. The dish can be customized with your favorite toppings, such as cheese, sour cream or avocado, for a delicious and comforting meal.

Prep Time / Cooking Time: 55 Minutes

Serving Size: 2 Persons

Ingredient List

- 1 lb. ground turkey
- 1 tablespoon olive oil
- 1 chopped onion
- 2 chopped red bell peppers
- 1 chopped green bell pepper
- 1 can (15 ounces) drained and rinsed kidney beans
- 1 can (14.5 ounces) undrained tomatoes
- 1 can (8 ounces) tomato sauce
- 1 teaspoon ground cumin
- 1 tablespoon chili powder
- 1/2 teaspoon garlic powder
- 1/2 teaspoon salt
- 1/4 teaspoon black pepper

XXXXXXXXXXXXXXXXX

Instructions

a) Heat the olive oil in a large pot over medium heat.

b) Stir in the turkey. Cook until browned.

c) Add the onion and bell peppers and cook them until they are tender.

d) Add the kidney beans, tomatoes, chili powder, cumin, tomato sauce, garlic powder, salt and black pepper to the pot.

e) Stir and bring to a boil.

f) Reduce the heat and simmer for 45 minutes, stirring occasionally.

g) Serve hot.

8. Shrimp and Broccoli Stir Fry

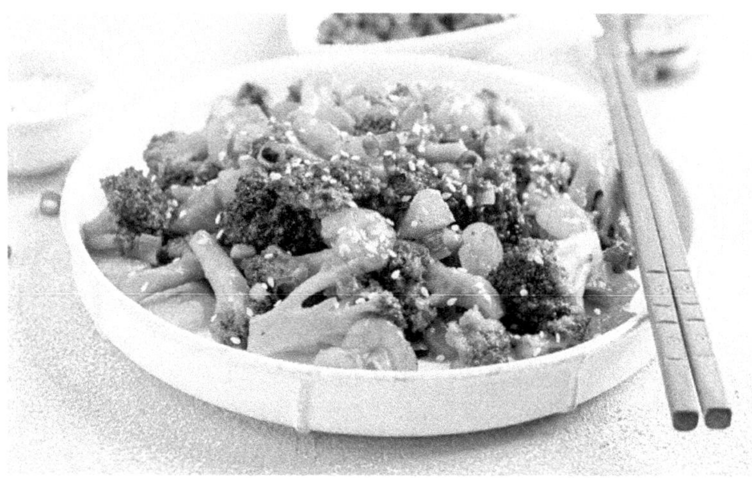

Shrimp and Broccoli Stir Fry is a quick and easy dish that is perfect for a healthy and flavorful dinner. It is made by stir-frying shrimp and broccoli in a savory sauce made with garlic, ginger and soy sauce. It is a great source of protein and nutrients and can be served over rice or noodles for a satisfying and delicious meal. The dish is easy to prepare and can be customized with your favorite toppings and add-ins.

Prep Time / Cooking Time: 55 Minutes

Serving Size: 2 Persons

Ingredient List

- 1 lb. peeled and deveined shrimp
- 2 cups broccoli florets
- 2 tablespoons vegetable oil
- 1 tablespoon minced garlic
- 1 tablespoon minced ginger
- 1/4 cup soy sauce
- 1/4 cup oyster sauce
- 1 tablespoon cornstarch
- 1/4 cup water

xxxxxxxxxxxxxxxxx

Instructions

a) Heat a pan over high heat and add the vegetable oil.

b) Add the ginger and garlic. Stir-fry for 10 seconds.

c) Add the shrimp, then stir-fry until pink, about 2-3 minutes.

d) Add the broccoli. Stir-fry for another 2-3 minutes.

e) In a small bowl, mix the oyster sauce, soy sauce, cornstarch and water.

f) Pour the sauce over the stir-fry and stir-fry until the sauce thickens, about 1-2 minutes.

g) Serve hot.

9. Mediterranean Chicken and Vegetable Skewers

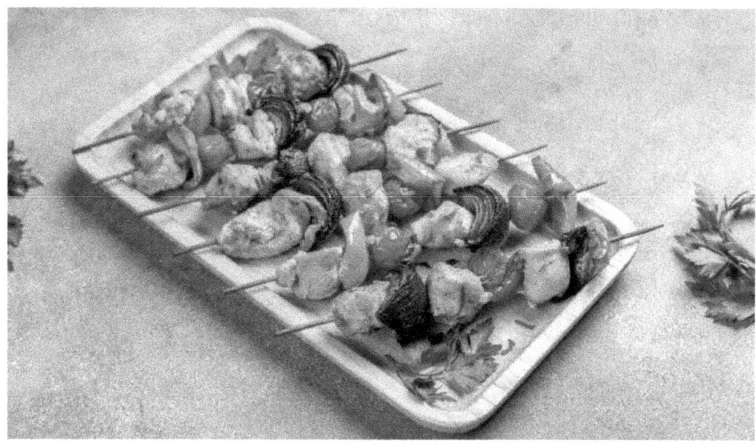

Mediterranean Chicken and Vegetable Skewers are a flavorful and healthy dish that is perfect for a summer barbecue or dinner party. They are made by marinating tender chicken and fresh vegetables, such as bell pepper, red onion and zucchini, in a blend of seasonings. The dish can be served with a side of hummus or tzatziki for a complete Mediterranean-inspired meal.

Prep Time / Cooking Time: 55 Minutes

Serving Size: 2 Persons

Ingredient List

- 2 sliced boneless chicken breasts
- 2 sliced red peppers
- 2 sliced yellow peppers
- 1 sliced red onion
- 2 sliced zucchinis
- 1/4 cup olive oil
- 2 tablespoons red wine vinegar
- 1 tablespoon dried oregano
- 1 teaspoon salt
- 1/2 teaspoon black pepper

XXXXXXXXXXXXXXXXX

Instructions

a) Preheat a grill to medium-high heat.

b) In a small bowl, whisk together the olive oil, red wine vinegar, oregano, salt and black pepper.

c) Thread the chicken breasts and vegetables onto skewers, alternating between each.

d) Brush the skewers with the mixture.

e) Grill for 10-12 minutes, turning occasionally, or until the chicken is cooked through and the vegetables are tender.

f) Serve hot and enjoy!

10. Spicy Peanut Tofu and Vegetable Stir Fry

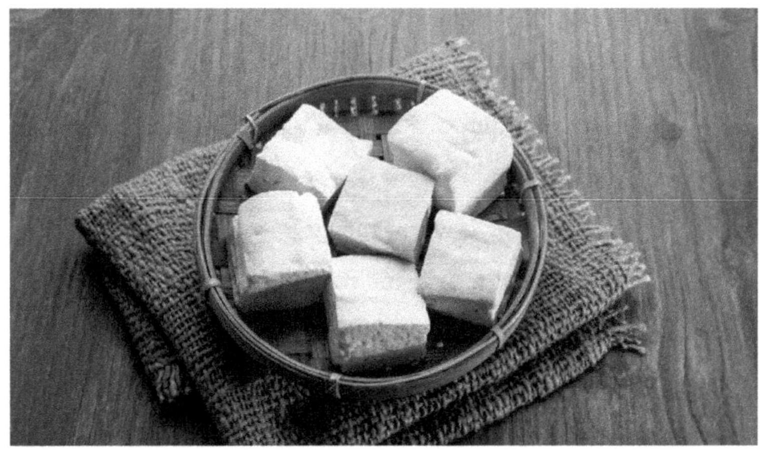

Spicy Peanut Tofu and Vegetable Stir Fry is a delicious and nutritious dish that is perfect for a meatless dinner option. It is made by stir-frying tofu and vegetables, such as bell pepper and broccoli, in a spicy peanut sauce. It is a great source of plant-based protein, fiber and fats, making it a satisfying and healthy meal. The dish can be served over rice or noodles for a complete and flavorful meal.

Prep Time / Cooking Time: 55 Minutes

Serving Size: 2 Persons

Ingredient List

- 1 tofu
- 1 red bell pepper
- 1 yellow bell pepper
- 1/2 red onion
- 1 cup broccoli florets
- 1/2 cup snow peas
- 1/4 cup peanuts
- 3 sliced garlic cloves
- 1 sliced ginger knot
- 2 tablespoons soy sauce
- 2 tablespoons peanut butter
- 1 tablespoon Sriracha sauce
- 1 tablespoon vegetable oil

XXXXXXXXXXXXXXXX

Instructions

a) Press the tofu to remove excess water and cut it into small cubes.

b) Cut the bell peppers and red onion into thin slices.

c) Heat a wok over medium-high heat and add the vegetable oil.

d) Add the garlic and ginger, then cook for 1 minute.

e) Add the tofu and cook it until it turns golden brown.

f) Add the bell pepper, red onion, broccoli and snow peas. Cook for 5-7 minutes or until the vegetables are tender.

g) In a small bowl, mix the soy sauce, peanut butter and Sriracha sauce.

h) Add the sauce to the wok and stir to coat it with the vegetables and tofu.

i) Serve topped with the peanuts.

11. Lentil Soup with Spinach and Tomatoes

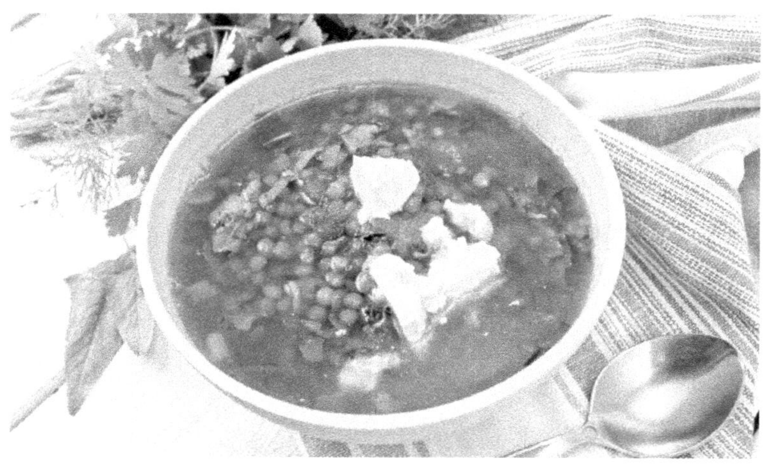

Lentil Soup with Spinach and Tomatoes is a comforting and nutritious dish that is perfect for a chilly day. The soup is made by simmering lentils with spinach, tomatoes and a blend of herbs and spices. It is a great source of protein, fiber and vitamins, making it a satisfying and healthy option. The dish can be served with a side of crusty bread for a complete and delicious meal.

Prep Time / Cooking Time: 55 Minutes

Serving Size: 2 Persons

Ingredient List

- 1 cup dried lentils
- 4 cups water
- 1 chopped onion
- 2 minced garlic cloves
- 5 ounces diced tomatoes
- 2 cups chopped fresh spinach
- 1 teaspoon cumin
- 1 teaspoon paprika
- Salt and pepper to taste

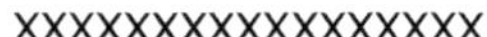

XXXXXXXXXXXXXXXXX

Instructions

a) Rinse the lentils and add them to a large pot with the water.

b) Add the onion and garlic.

c) Bring to a boil, then reduce the heat to simmer. Cover and cook for 30 minutes.

d) Add the tomatoes, cumin, paprika and salt and pepper to the pot.

e) Cover and continue to simmer for an additional 15 minutes.

f) Add the spinach to the pot. Cook for an additional 10 minutes.

g) Serve hot and enjoy!

12. Baked Cod with Tomatoes and Olives

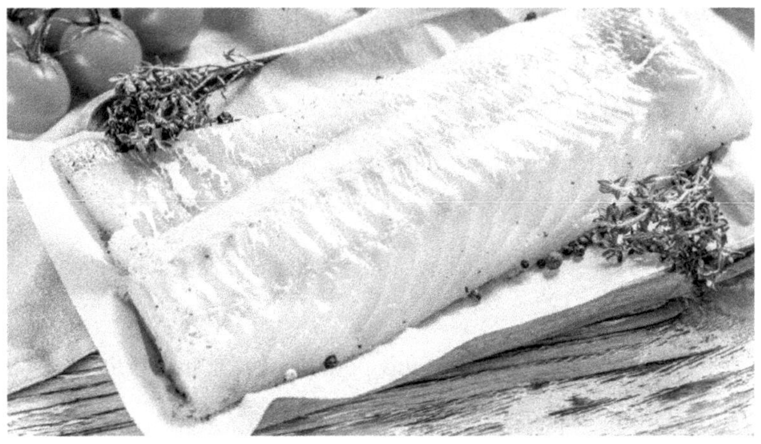

Baked Cod with Tomatoes and Olives is a flavorful and healthy dish that is perfect for a quick and easy dinner. It is made by baking cod fillets with cherry tomatoes, olives and garlic. It is a great source of protein and fats, making it a satisfying and nutritious option. The dish can be served with a side of roasted vegetables or a simple salad for a complete and delicious meal.

Prep Time / Cooking Time: 55 Minutes

Serving Size: 2 Persons

Ingredient List

- 2 cod fillets
- 1 cup halved cherry tomatoes
- 1/4 cup sliced olives
- 2 minced garlic cloves
- 2 tablespoons olive oil
- 1/2 teaspoon salt
- 1/4 teaspoon black pepper

xxxxxxxxxxxxxxxxx

Instructions

a) Preheat the oven to 375°F.

b) In a mixing bowl, combine the cherry tomatoes, olives, garlic, olive oil, salt and black pepper.

c) Place the cod fillets in a baking dish.

d) Pour the mixture over the fish.

e) Bake for 40-45 minutes or until the fish is cooked through and flakes easily with a fork.

f) Serve hot and enjoy!

13. Quinoa Fried Rice with Vegetables and Shrimp

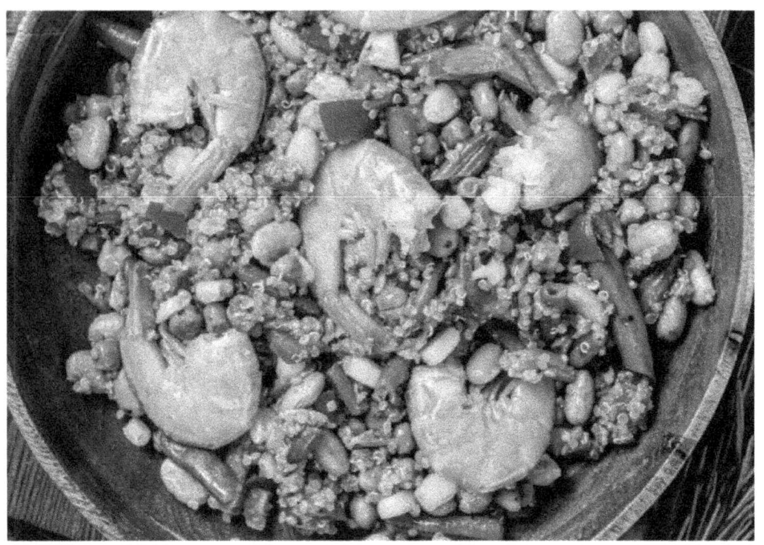

Quinoa Fried Rice with Vegetables and Shrimp is a healthy and delicious twist on a classic dish. It replaces traditional rice with quinoa, a protein-rich grain, and adds vegetables, such as bell pepper and onion, and tender shrimp. It is a great source of protein, fiber and nutrients, making it a satisfying and nutritious meal. The dish can be customized with your favorite toppings and add-ins for a flavorful and healthy meal.

Prep Time / Cooking Time: 55 Minutes

Serving Size: 2 Persons

Ingredient List

- 1 tablespoon olive oil
- 1/2 cup quinoa
- 1 cup water
- 1/2 chopped onion
- 1/2 chopped red bell pepper
- 1/2 cup frozen peas
- 1/2 cup frozen corn
- 1/2 cup cooked shrimp
- 2 minced garlic cloves
- 2 beaten eggs
- 2 tablespoons soy sauce
- 1/4 teaspoon salt
- 1/4 teaspoon black pepper

XXXXXXXXXXXXXXXX

Instructions

a) Rinse the quinoa in a fine mesh strainer and place it in a medium pot with the water. Bring to a boil, cover and simmer for 15 minutes. Remove from the heat and let stand for 5 minutes.

b) Heat the olive oil in a large skillet over medium heat. Add the onion and red bell pepper, then cook for 3-4 minutes until softened.

c) Add the peas, corn, shrimp and garlic to the skillet. Cook for 2-3 minutes until heated through.

d) Push the vegetables and shrimp on the side of the skillet and add the eggs to the other side. Scramble the eggs with a spatula until cooked through.

e) Add the quinoa to the skillet and stir it to combine it with the vegetables, shrimp and eggs.

f) Add the soy sauce, salt and black pepper to the skillet. Then, stir to coat all ingredients evenly.

g) Cook for an additional 2-3 minutes until heated through.

h) Serve hot and enjoy!

14. Chicken and Broccoli Alfredo

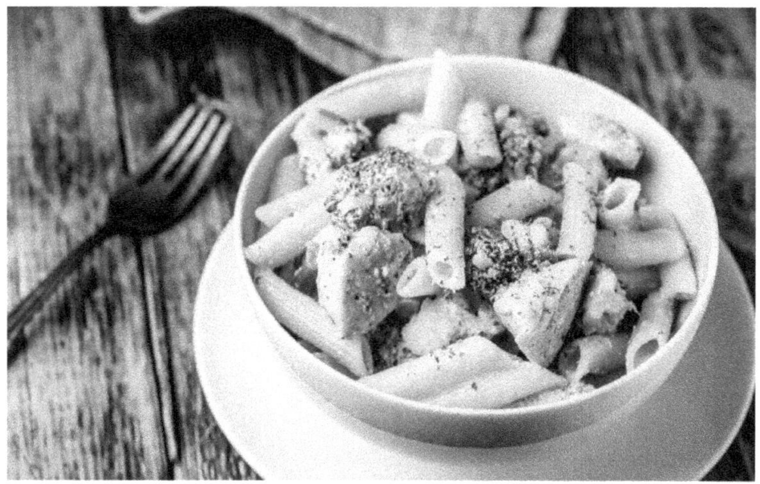

Chicken and Broccoli Alfredo is a classic and comforting dish that is perfect for a cozy night in. It is made by sautéing chicken and broccoli in a creamy Alfredo sauce made with butter, heavy cream and Parmesan cheese. It is a great source of protein and calcium, making it a satisfying and delicious meal. The dish can be served over your favorite pasta for a complete and comforting meal.

Prep Time / Cooking Time: 55 Minutes

Serving Size: 2 Persons

Ingredient List

- 8 ounces fettuccine pasta
- 2 chicken breasts
- 2 cups broccoli florets
- 2 tablespoons butter, divided
- 2 garlic cloves
- 1/2 cup grated parmesan cheese
- 1 cup heavy cream
- Salt and pepper to taste

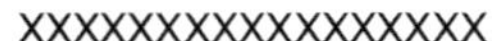

XXXXXXXXXXXXXXXX

Instructions

a) Cook the fettuccine pasta according to the package instructions in a large pot of salted boiling water and drain and set it aside.

b) Cut the chicken breasts into bite-sized pieces and season them to taste. Heat 1 tablespoon of the butter in a skillet over medium-high heat and cook the chicken until browned and cooked through. Then, remove from the pan and put aside.

c) In the same skillet, melt the remaining butter and sauté the garlic until fragrant. Add the broccoli, then cook until tender; take out from the skillet and set aside.

d) In the same skillet, whisk together the heavy cream and parmesan cheese until the cheese is melted and the sauce is smooth. Season to taste.

e) Add the pasta, chicken and broccoli to the skillet with the sauce. Toss until everything is coated in the Alfredo sauce.

f) Serve hot and enjoy!

15. Greek Yogurt Chicken Salad

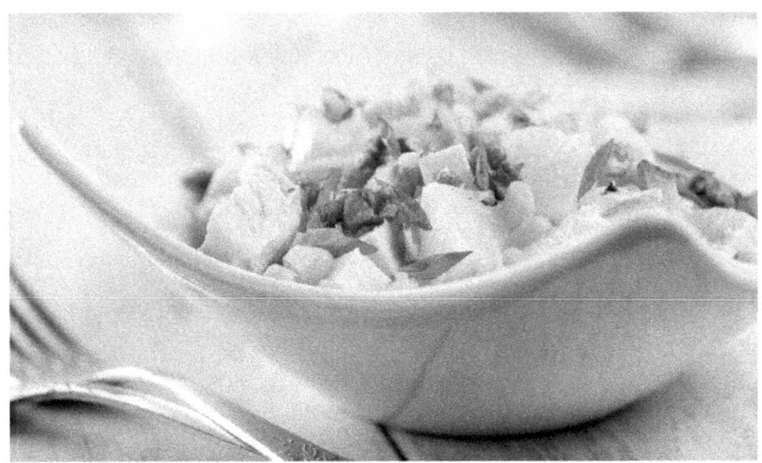

Greek Yogurt Chicken Salad is a healthy and delicious twist on a classic dish. It replaces traditional mayonnaise with creamy Greek yogurt and adds fresh vegetables, such as celery and red onion, and tender chicken. It is a great source of protein and calcium, making it a satisfying and nutritious meal. The dish can be served on a bed of greens or in a sandwich for a complete and delicious meal.

Prep Time / Cooking Time: 55 Minutes

Serving Size: 2 Persons

Ingredient List

- 2 boneless and skinless chicken breasts
- 1/2 cup plain Greek yogurt
- 1/4 cup diced red onion
- 1/4 cup diced celery
- 1/4 cup diced apple
- 1/4 cup chopped walnuts
- 1 tablespoon lemon juice
- 1/2 teaspoon garlic powder
- Salt and pepper to taste

XXXXXXXXXXXXXXXXX

Instructions

a) Preheat the oven to 375°F (190°C).

b) Place the chicken breasts on a baking sheet and season them with garlic powder and salt and pepper. Bake for 25-30 minutes or until cooked through.

c) Let the chicken cool for 5 minutes, then shred it using a fork.

d) In a mixing bowl, combine the chicken, Greek yogurt, red onion, celery, apple, walnuts, lemon juice and salt and pepper. Mix well.

e) Chill the salad in the refrigerator for at least 30 minutes before serving it.

16. Baked Lemon Herb Chicken with Roasted Vegetables

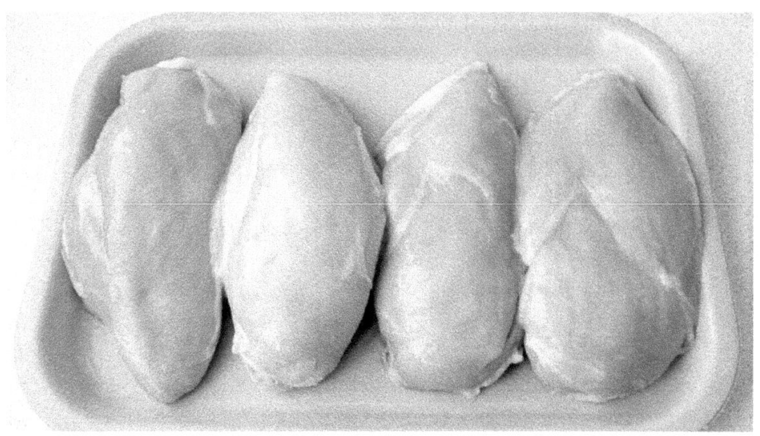

Baked Lemon Herb Chicken with Roasted Vegetables is a flavorful and healthy dish that is perfect for a busy weeknight. It is made by marinating tender chicken in a tangy lemon herb sauce and then baking it with fresh vegetables. It is a great source of protein, fiber and vitamins, making it a satisfying and nutritious option. The dish can be served with a side of brown rice or quinoa for a complete and delicious meal.

Prep Time / Cooking Time: 55 Minutes

Serving Size: 2 Persons

Ingredient List

- 2 chicken breasts
- 1 lemon
- 1 teaspoon dried thyme
- 1 teaspoon dried rosemary
- 1 teaspoon dried oregano
- 1 teaspoon garlic powder
- 1/2 teaspoon salt
- 1/4 teaspoon black pepper
- 2 tablespoons olive oil
- 2 cups mixed vegetables (carrot, broccoli and cauliflower)
- 1 tablespoon balsamic vinegar

XXXXXXXXXXXXXXXX

Instructions

a) Preheat the oven to 375°F.

b) Combine the thyme, oregano, rosemary, garlic powder, salt and black pepper in a small bowl.

c) Place the chicken breasts in a baking dish and coat them with the olive oil.

d) Sprinkle the mixture over the chicken and squeeze the lemon juice over the top.

e) Bake for 35-40 minutes or until the chicken is cooked through.

f) Meanwhile, chop the vegetables into bite-sized pieces and place them in a mixing bowl.

g) Drizzle with the balsamic vinegar and toss to coat.

h) Spread the vegetables out on a baking sheet and roast them in the oven for 15-20 minutes or until tender.

i) Serve the chicken with the vegetables on the side.

17. Sweet Potato and Black Bean Enchilada

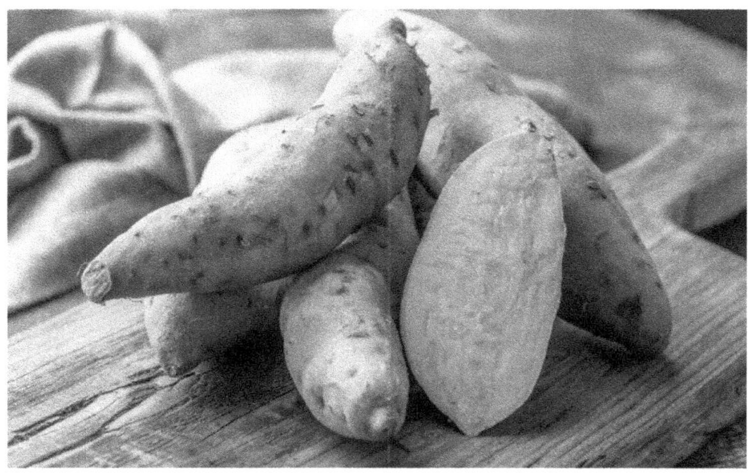

Sweet Potato and Black Bean Enchilada is a delicious and healthy twist on a traditional enchilada. This hearty dish features roasted sweet potato and black beans, rolled up in corn tortillas and smothered in a spicy tomato sauce and melted cheese. It is a flavorful and satisfying dish that is perfect for weeknight dinners or potlucks. The enchilada is also vegetarian and gluten-free, making it a great choice for anyone with dietary restrictions or looking for a meatless meal option.

Prep Time / Cooking Time: 55 Minutes

Serving Size: 2 Persons

Ingredient List

- 2 peeled and cubed medium sweet potatoes
- 15 ounces drained and rinsed black beans
- 1/2 diced onion
- 2 minced garlic cloves
- 1 tablespoon olive oil
- 1 teaspoon cumin
- 1/2 teaspoon chili powder
- 1/2 teaspoon paprika
- 1/4 teaspoon salt
- 4-6 corn tortillas
- 1/2 cup shredded cheddar cheese
- 1/4 cup chopped fresh cilantro

XXXXXXXXXXXXXXXXX

Instructions

a) Preheat the oven to 375°F.

b) In a frying pan over medium heat, cook the onion and garlic in the olive oil until softened.

c) Add the black beans, sweet potatoes, cumin, chili powder, paprika and salt to the pan. Then, cook for 10-15 minutes until the sweet potatoes are tender.

d) Warm the corn tortillas in the microwave or on a griddle.

e) In a mixing bowl, mix the mixture with the cilantro.

f) Fill each tortilla with the mixture, then roll up.

g) Place the tortillas seam-side down in a baking dish.

h) Sprinkle the cheddar cheese over the top of the enchiladas.

i) Bake for 20-25 minutes or until the cheese is melted and bubbly.

18. Creamy Tomato Soup with Grilled Cheese Croutons

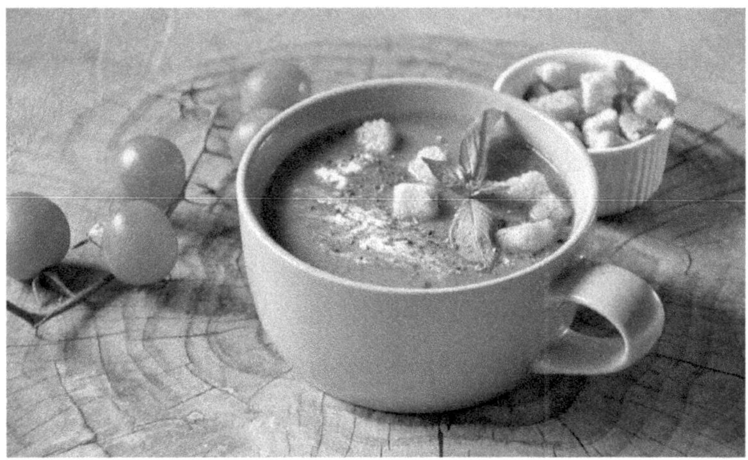

Creamy Tomato Soup with Grilled Cheese Croutons is a classic and comforting dish that is perfect for a cozy night in. It is made with tomatoes and heavy cream for a rich and flavorful taste. It is served with grilled cheese croutons, made by toasting bread with cheese, for a delicious and satisfying meal. The dish is a great source of vitamins and calcium, making it a nutritious and delicious option.

Prep Time / Cooking Time: 55 Minutes

Serving Size: 2 Persons

Ingredient List

- 2 cans whole peeled tomatoes
- 1 onion
- 3 garlic cloves
- 2 cups chicken broth
- 1/4 cup heavy cream
- 4 bread slices
- 4 cheddar cheese slices
- 2 tablespoons butter

XXXXXXXXXXXXXXXXX

Instructions

a) Preheat a pan to medium heat.

b) Add the onion and garlic to the pan. Cook until the onion is translucent.

c) Add the tomatoes and chicken broth and bring to a simmer.

d) Simmer for 30 minutes.

e) Remove from the heat and let cool for a few minutes.

f) Pour the mixture into the blender and blend until smooth.

g) Return to the pot and stir in the heavy cream.

h) Preheat a pan over medium heat.

i) Spread the butter on one side of each bread slice.

j) Place the bread butter-side down in the pan and top it with the cheddar cheese.

k) Cook until the cheese is melted and the bread is golden brown.

l) Cut into small squares to use as croutons.

m) Serve the soup with the croutons.

19. Grilled Shrimp Taco with Avocado Salsa

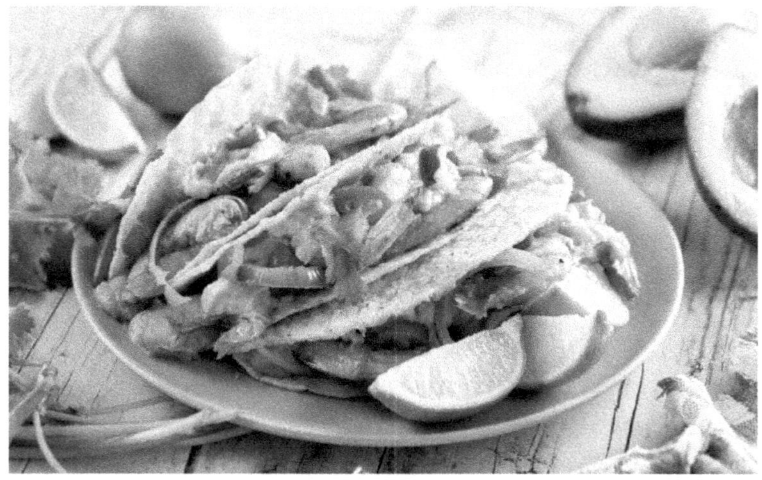

Grilled Shrimp Taco with Avocado Salsa is a fresh and flavorful dish that is perfect for a summer dinner. It is made by marinating tender shrimp in a blend of spices, grilling it to perfection and serving it in warm corn tortillas with a fresh avocado salsa. It is a great source of protein and fats, making it a satisfying and nutritious option. The dish can be customized with your favorite toppings for a delicious and personalized meal.

Prep Time / Cooking Time: 55 Minutes

Serving Size: 2 Persons

Ingredient List

- 1/2 lb. peeled and deveined large shrimp
- 2 tablespoons olive oil
- 1/4 teaspoon black pepper
- 1/4 teaspoon salt
- 1/4 teaspoon garlic powder
- 1/2 diced avocado
- 1/4 cup diced red onion
- 1/4 cup chopped fresh cilantro
- 1 juiced lime
- 4 small corn tortillas

XXXXXXXXXXXXXXXXX

Instructions

a) Preheat a grill to medium-high heat.

b) In a mixing bowl, combine the shrimp, olive oil, salt, black pepper and garlic powder. Toss to coat.

c) Grill the shrimp for 2-3 minutes per side or until cooked through.

d) In a separate mixing bowl, combine the avocado, red onion, cilantro and lime juice. Toss to combine.

e) Warm the corn tortillas on the grill for 30 seconds per side.

f) Assemble the taco by placing the shrimp on each tortilla and topping it with the avocado salsa.

20. Broiled Salmon with Asparagus and Lemon Butter

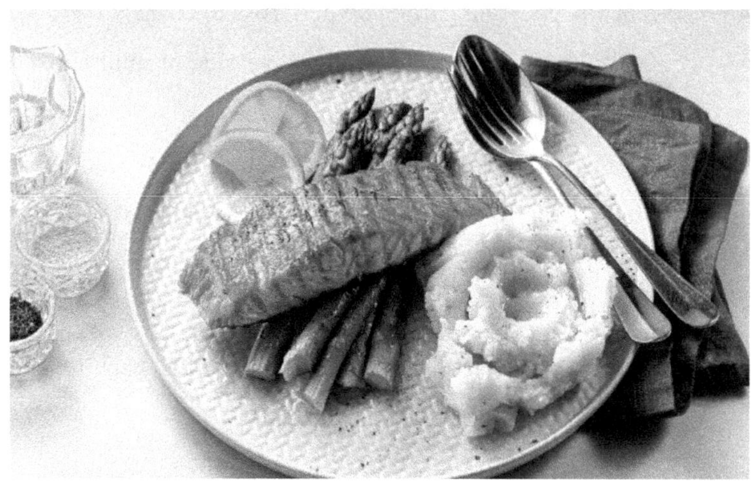

Broiled Salmon with Asparagus and Lemon Butter is a healthy and flavorful dish that is perfect for a quick and easy dinner. It is made by broiling salmon and asparagus with a tangy lemon butter sauce for a delicious and satisfying taste. It is a great source of protein, omega-3 fatty acids and vitamins, making it a nutritious and delicious option. The dish can be served with a side of brown rice or quinoa for a complete and delicious meal.

Prep Time / Cooking Time: 55 Minutes

Serving Size: 2 Persons

Ingredient List

- 2 salmon fillets
- 1 pound asparagus
- 4 tablespoons unsalted butter, divided
- 1 lemon
- Salt and pepper to taste

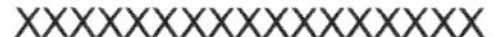

Instructions

a) Preheat the broiler to high heat.

b) Line a baking sheet with aluminum foil.

c) Rinse the salmon and pat it dry with a paper towel.

d) Place the fish on the baking sheet and season it to taste.

e) Broil for 10-12 minutes or until cooked through.

f) While the fish is cooking, prepare the asparagus by rinsing and trimming the ends.

g) Melt 2 tablespoons of the butter in a skillet over medium heat.

h) Add the asparagus to the skillet. Then, season to taste.

i) Cook for 8-10 minutes or until tender.

j) While the asparagus is cooking, prepare the lemon butter by melting the remaining butter in a small saucepan.

k) Squeeze the lemon juice into the saucepan and stir to combine.

l) Remove the fish from the heat and serve it with the asparagus and lemon butter sauce.

21. Zucchini Noodles with Pesto and Shrimp

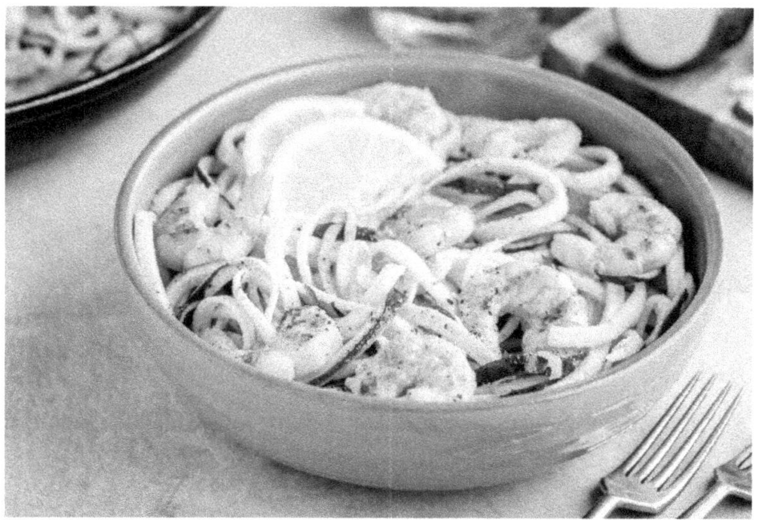

Zucchini Noodles with Pesto and Shrimp are a light and healthy dish that is perfect for a summer lunch or dinner. The dish is made by spiralizing zucchini into noodles and serving them with a homemade pesto sauce and shrimp. It is a great source of protein and vitamins, making it a satisfying and nutritious option. It can be customized with your favorite toppings and add-ins for a flavorful and healthy meal.

Prep Time / Cooking Time: 55 Minutes

Serving Size: 2 Persons

Ingredient List

- 2 spiralized medium zucchini
- 1/2 lb. peeled and deveined shrimp
- 2 tablespoons olive oil
- 1/4 cup pesto
- Salt and pepper to taste

XXXXXXXXXXXXXXXX

Instructions

a) Heat the olive oil in a pan over medium heat.

b) Add the shrimp. Cook for 3-5 minutes per side or until ready.

c) Remove from the heat and set aside.

d) Add the zucchini. Cook for 2-3 minutes or until slightly softened.

e) Add the pesto and stir it to combine with the zucchini.

f) Add the shrimp back to the pan. Then, stir to combine with the zucchini and pesto.

g) Season to taste.

h) Serve immediately.

22. Slow Cooker Chicken and Vegetable Soup

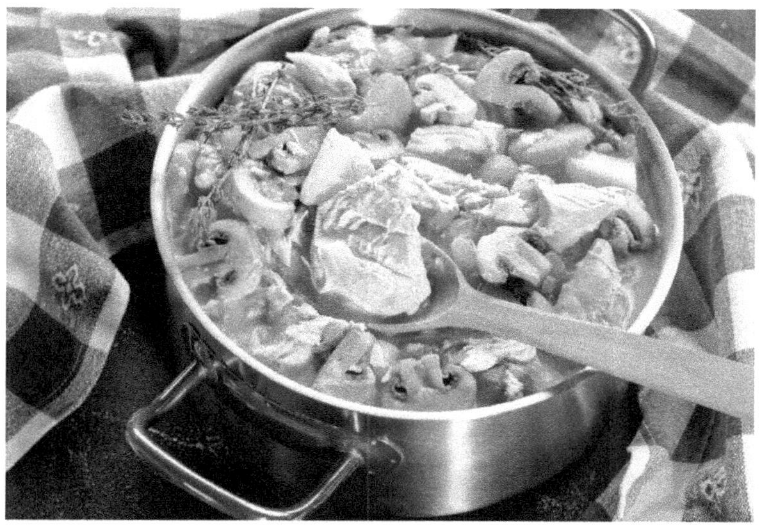

Slow Cooker Chicken and Vegetable Soup is a comforting and healthy soup that is perfect for chilly days. This recipe features tender chicken, a variety of fresh vegetables and flavorful seasonings, all simmered together in a slow cooker for maximum flavor and convenience. The result is a warm and hearty soup that is perfect for lunch or dinner and can be customized with any vegetables you have on hand. It is an easy and nutritious meal that will warm you up from the inside out.

Prep Time / Cooking Time: 55 Minutes

Serving Size: 2 Persons

Ingredient List

- 2 chicken breasts
- 4 cups chicken broth
- 1 onion
- 3 garlic cloves
- 3 carrots
- 2 celery stalks
- 1 teaspoon dried thyme
- 1 teaspoon dried oregano
- 1 teaspoon salt
- 1/2 teaspoon black pepper
- 2 cups chopped kale

XXXXXXXXXXXXXXXXX

Instructions

a) Place the chicken breasts, chicken broth, onion, garlic, carrots, celery, thyme, oregano, salt and black pepper in the slow cooker.

b) Cook on low for 8 hours or high for 4 hours.

c) Take the chicken out and shred it with 2 forks.

d) Return the chicken to the slow cooker and add the kale.

e) Cook for an additional 15 minutes on high.

f) Serve hot and enjoy!

23. Roasted Butternut Squash and Brussels Sprout Salad

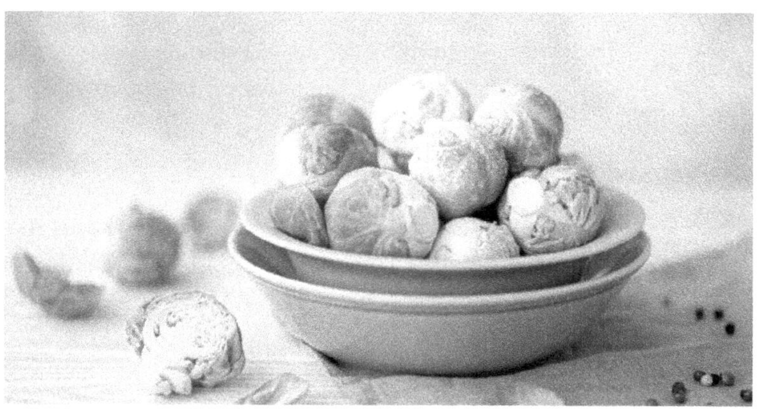

Roasted Butternut Squash and Brussels Sprout Salad is a delicious and healthy dish that is perfect for a fall dinner. It is made by roasting butternut squash and Brussels sprouts and serving them over a bed of greens with a tangy vinaigrette dressing. It is a great source of fiber, vitamins and fats, making it a nutritious and satisfying option. The dish can be customized with your favorite toppings for a flavorful and healthy meal.

Prep Time / Cooking Time: 55 Minutes

Serving Size: 2 Persons

Ingredient List

For the Salad:

- 1 peeled and cubed small butternut squash
- 1/2 lb. trimmed and halved Brussels sprouts
- 2 tablespoons olive oil
- 1/4 teaspoon salt
- 1/4 teaspoon black pepper
- 2 cups mixed greens
- 1/4 cup crumbled feta cheese
- 1/4 cup dried cranberries
- 1/4 cup chopped pecans
- 1/4 cup crumbled feta cheese

For the Dressing:

- 2 tablespoons lemon juice
- 1 tablespoon honey
- 1/4 cup olive oil
- Salt and pepper to taste

XXXXXXXXXXXXXXXXX

Instructions

a) Preheat the oven to 400°F (200°C).

b) In a mixing bowl, combine the olive oil, Brussels sprouts, butternut squash, salt and black pepper.

c) Spread the vegetables onto a baking sheet.

d) Roast for 35-40 minutes or until tender and lightly browned.

e) In a small bowl, whisk together the olive oil, lemon juice, honey and salt and black pepper.

f) In a serving bowl, combine the mixed greens, vegetables, feta cheese, pecans and cranberries.

g) Drizzle the dressing over the salad and toss to combine.

h) Serve and enjoy!

24. Easy Quinoa and Vegetable Stuffed Pepper

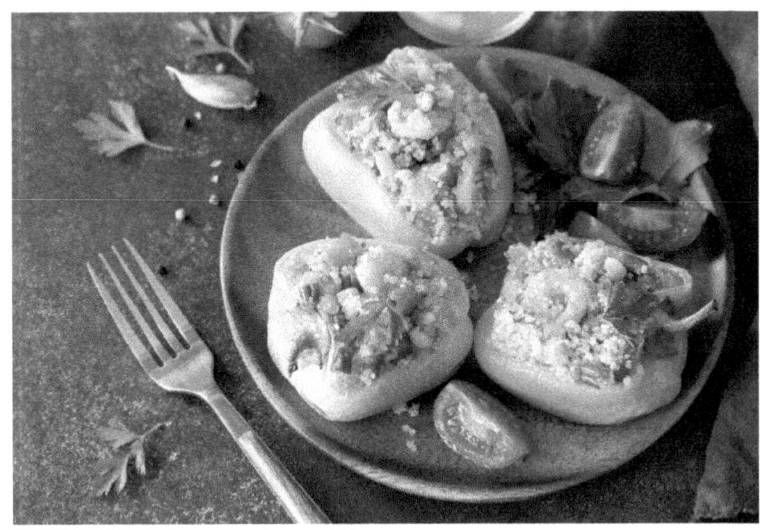

Easy Quinoa and Vegetable Stuffed Pepper is a healthy and flavorful dish that is perfect for a vegetarian dinner. It is made by stuffing bell peppers with a mixture of quinoa, vegetables and spices and baking them to perfection. It is a great source of protein, fiber and vitamins, making it a nutritious and delicious option. The dish can be customized with your favorite toppings and add-ins for a flavorful and healthy meal.

Prep Time / Cooking Time: 55 Minutes

Serving Size: 2 Persons

Ingredient List

- 2 bell peppers
- 1/2 cup quinoa
- 1 cup vegetable broth
- 1/2 chopped onion
- 1 minced garlic clove
- 1/2 cup drained and rinsed black beans
- 1/2 cup corn
- 1/2 cup diced tomatoes
- 1/2 teaspoon cumin
- 1/2 teaspoon chili powder
- 1/4 cup shredded cheddar cheese

XXXXXXXXXXXXXXXX

Instructions

a) Preheat the oven to 375°F.

b) Cut the tops of the bell peppers and remove the seeds and membranes.

c) In a medium saucepan, bring the quinoa and vegetable broth to a boil over medium-high heat. Reduce the heat to low and simmer for 15-20 minutes or until the quinoa is cooked and the liquid is absorbed.

d) In a large skillet, sauté the garlic and onion until softened. Add the black beans, corn, tomatoes, cumin and chili powder. Cook for 5-7 minutes or until heated through.

e) Add the quinoa to the skillet, then stir to combine.

f) Stuff the bell peppers with the mixture. Place in a baking dish.

g) Bake for 25-30 minutes or until the bell peppers are soft and the filling is heated.

h) Sprinkle the cheddar cheese over the top of each bell pepper. Bake for 5-7 minutes or until the cheese is melted and bubbly.

25. Vegan Lentil Soup

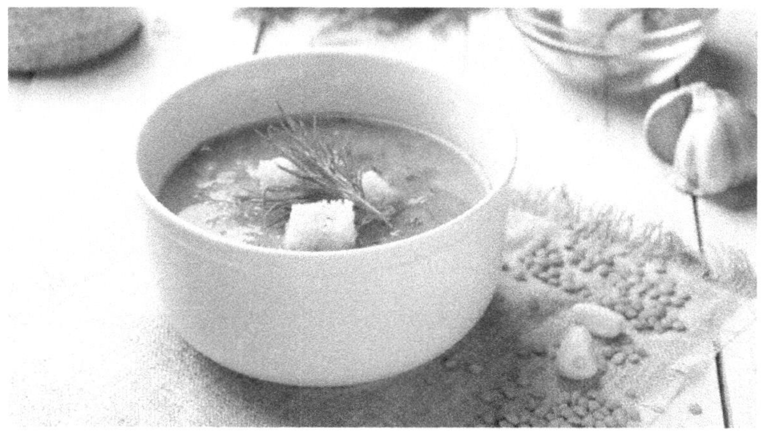

Vegan Lentil Soup is a hearty and nutritious soup made with red lentils and herbs. It is a perfect dish for vegans and vegetarians, as it is rich in protein, fiber and other nutrients. The soup is usually cooked in vegetable broth and seasoned with a variety of spices, such as cumin and turmeric. It is a simple and delicious dish that can be enjoyed all year round.

Prep Time / Cooking Time: 55 Minutes

Serving Size: 2 Persons

Ingredient List

- 1 cup red lentils
- 4 cups vegetable broth
- 1 chopped onion
- 2 minced garlic cloves
- 1 chopped carrot
- 1 chopped celery stalk
- 1 teaspoon cumin
- 1 teaspoon paprika
- 1/2 teaspoon turmeric
- 1/4 teaspoon cayenne pepper
- 2 tablespoons olive oil
- Salt and pepper to taste

XXXXXXXXXXXXXXXX

Instructions

a) Rinse the red lentils in cold water and drain them.

b) In a large pot over medium heat, heat the olive oil.

c) Add the onion. Cook for 7 minutes until crystalline.

d) Add the garlic. Cook for 1 minute.

e) Add the carrot and celery and cook them for 7 minutes until they soften.

f) Add the cumin, paprika, turmeric and cayenne pepper and cook for 1 minute.

g) Add the vegetable broth and lentils to the pot. Then, bring to a boil.

h) Reduce the heat to low and simmer for 40 minutes until the lentils are tender.

i) Season to taste.

j) Serve hot and enjoy!

26. Spinach and Feta Stuffed Chicken Breast

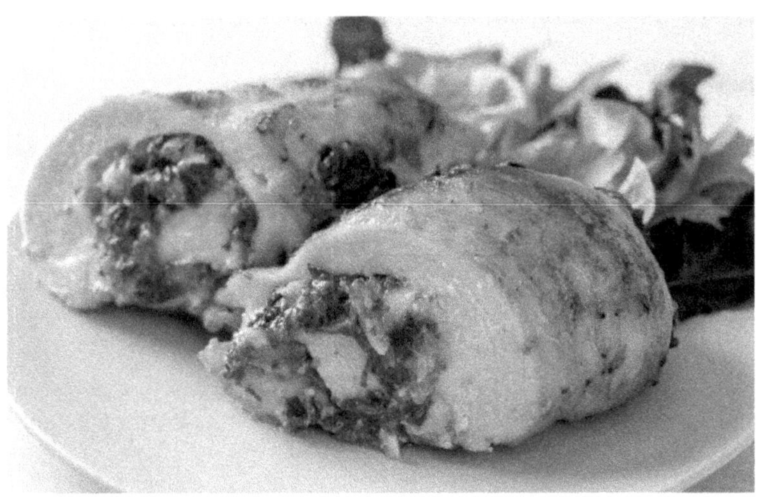

Spinach and Feta Stuffed Chicken Breast is a flavorful and healthy dish that is perfect for a special occasion or a fancy dinner. It is made by stuffing chicken breasts with a mixture of spinach, feta cheese and garlic and baking them to perfection. It is a great source of protein and calcium, making it a satisfying and delicious meal. The dish can be served with a side of roasted vegetables or a simple salad for a complete and delicious meal.

Prep Time / Cooking Time: 55 Minutes

Serving Size: 2 Persons

Ingredient List

- 2 boneless and skinless chicken breasts
- 1 cup chopped spinach
- 1/2 cup crumbled feta cheese
- 1/4 cup breadcrumbs
- 1/4 teaspoon garlic powder
- 1/4 teaspoon salt
- 1/4 teaspoon black pepper
- 2 tablespoons olive oil

XXXXXXXXXXXXXXXX

Instructions

a) Preheat the oven to 375°F (190°C).

b) In a mixing bowl, combine the spinach, feta cheese, breadcrumbs, garlic powder, salt and black pepper.

c) Butterfly the chicken breasts by slicing them horizontally, but not all the way through, and open them like a book.

d) Place a spoonful of the mixture on one side of each chicken breast, then fold the other side over the mixture.

e) Use toothpicks to secure the chicken breasts closed.

f) Heat the olive oil in a large oven-safe skillet over medium-high heat.

g) Add the chicken to the skillet. Then, cook for 2-3 minutes on each side or until browned.

h) Transfer the skillet to the oven and bake for 30-35 minutes or until the chicken is cooked through and no longer pink in the center.

i) Remove the toothpicks before serving.

j) Enjoy!

27. Roasted Vegetable and Quinoa Salad

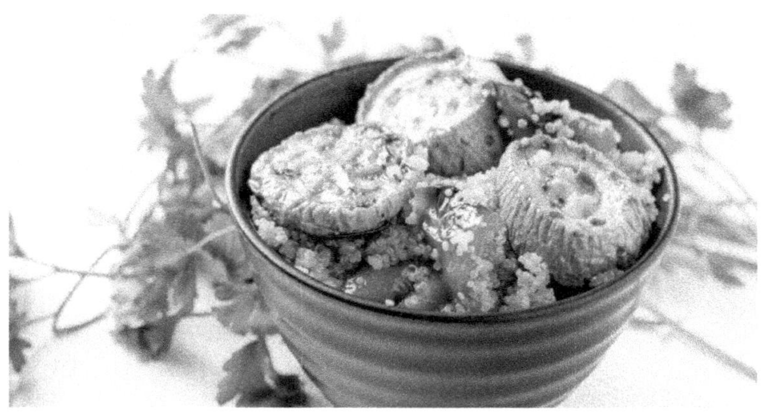

Roasted Vegetable and Quinoa Salad is a healthy and flavorful dish that is perfect for a light lunch or dinner. It is made by roasting vegetables, such as bell pepper, zucchini and red onion, and serving them over a bed of quinoa with a tangy vinaigrette dressing. It is a great source of protein, fiber and vitamins, making it a satisfying and nutritious option. The dish can be customized with your favorite toppings and add-ins for a flavorful and healthy meal.

Prep Time / Cooking Time: 55 Minutes

Serving Size: 2 Persons

Ingredient List

- 1 cup quinoa
- 2 cups chopped mixed vegetables (bell peppers, zucchini and red onion)
- 2 tablespoons olive oil, divided
- Salt and pepper to taste
- 2 cups mixed greens
- 1/4 cup crumbled feta cheese
- 1/4 cup chopped fresh herbs (parsley and basil)
- 2 tablespoons balsamic vinegar

XXXXXXXXXXXXXXXXX

Instructions

a) Preheat the oven to 400°F.

b) In a saucepan, cook the quinoa according to the package instructions.

c) On a baking sheet, toss the mixed vegetables with 1 tablespoon of the olive oil and salt and pepper. Roast for 25-30 minutes or until tender and lightly browned.

d) In a mixing bowl, whisk together the balsamic vinegar and the remaining olive oil to make the dressing.

e) Add the quinoa, vegetables, mixed greens, feta cheese and herbs to the mixing bowl with the dressing. Toss to combine.

f) Divide the salad into 2 bowls and serve.

28. Greek Chicken Bowl with Roasted Vegetables and Lemon Tahini Sauce

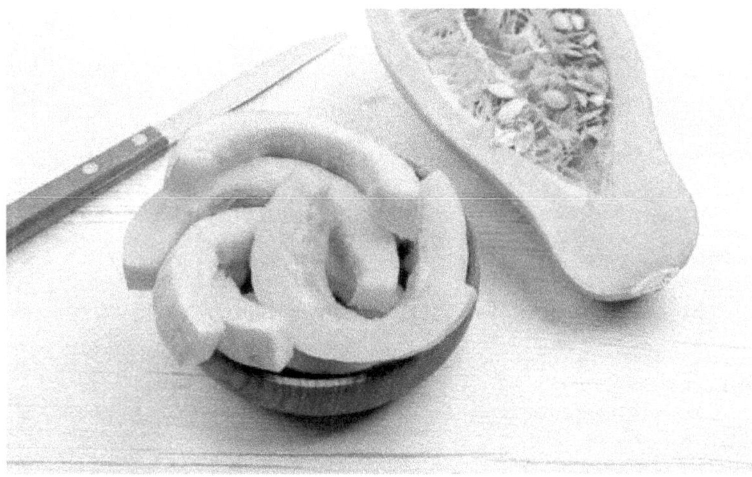

Greek Chicken Bowl with Roasted Vegetables and Lemon Tahini Sauce is a flavorful and healthy dish that is perfect for meal prep or a quick and easy dinner. It is made by roasting chicken and vegetables and serving them with a tangy lemon tahini sauce. The dish is a great source of protein, fiber and fats, making it a satisfying and nutritious option.

Prep Time / Cooking Time: 55 Minutes

Serving Size: 2 Persons

Ingredient List

For the Roasted Vegetables:

- 1 seeded and sliced red bell pepper
- 1 seeded and sliced yellow bell pepper
- 1 sliced red onion
- 1 sliced zucchini
- 1 sliced yellow squash
- 2 tablespoons olive oil
- 1/2 teaspoon dried oregano
- 1/2 teaspoon garlic powder
- 1/4 teaspoon salt

For the Chicken:

- 2 boneless and skinless chicken breasts
- 1 tablespoon olive oil
- 1/2 teaspoon dried oregano
- 1/2 teaspoon garlic powder
- 1/4 teaspoon salt

For the Lemon Tahini Sauce:

- 1/4 cup tahini
- 2 tablespoons lemon juice
- 2 tablespoons water

- 1 minced garlic clove
- 1/4 teaspoon salt

XXXXXXXXXXXXXXXXX

Instructions

a) Preheat the oven to 400°F.

b) In a mixing bowl, toss together the bell peppers, red onion, zucchini and yellow squash with the olive oil, oregano, garlic powder and salt. Spread the vegetables out on a baking sheet in a single layer.

c) Bake for 25 minutes, stirring once halfway through.

d) Meanwhile, heat a grill pan over medium-high heat. Brush the chicken breasts with the olive oil and season them with the oregano, garlic powder and salt. Grill the chicken for 6-8 minutes per side or until cooked through.

e) In a small mixing bowl, whisk together the tahini, lemon juice, water, garlic and salt to make the lemon tahini sauce.

f) To assemble the bowl, divide the vegetables and chicken between 2 bowls. Drizzle each bowl with the lemon tahini sauce.

g) Serve immediately.

29. One-Pan Balsamic Chicken with Roasted Vegetables

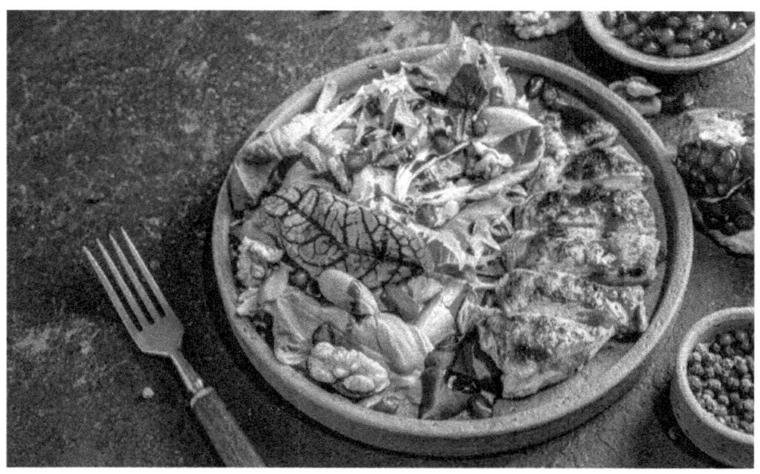

One-Pan Balsamic Chicken with Roasted Vegetables is a flavorful and easy dish that is perfect for a busy weeknight. It is made by marinating tender chicken in a tangy balsamic sauce and then roasting it with fresh vegetables. It is a great source of protein, fiber and vitamins, making it a satisfying and healthy option. The dish can be served with a side of quinoa or brown rice for a complete and delicious meal.

Prep Time / Cooking Time: 55 Minutes

Serving Size: 2 Persons

Ingredient List

- 2 boneless without skin chicken breasts
- 1 sliced red bell pepper
- 1 sliced yellow bell pepper
- 1 sliced zucchini
- 1 sliced red onion
- 2 tablespoons olive oil
- 1/4 cup balsamic vinegar
- 1 tablespoon honey
- 2 minced garlic cloves
- 1 tablespoon dried basil
- Salt and pepper to taste

XXXXXXXXXXXXXXXXX

Instructions

a) Preheat the oven to 400°F (200°C).

b) In a mixing bowl, whisk together the olive oil, balsamic vinegar, honey, garlic, basil and salt and pepper.

c) Place the chicken breasts on a baking sheet and coat them with half of the mixture.

d) Arrange the vegetables around the chicken on the baking sheet and coat them with the remaining mixture.

e) Bake for 40-45 minutes or until the chicken is cooked through and the vegetables are tender.

f) Serve hot and enjoy!

30. Cauliflower Fried Rice with Vegetables and Shrimp

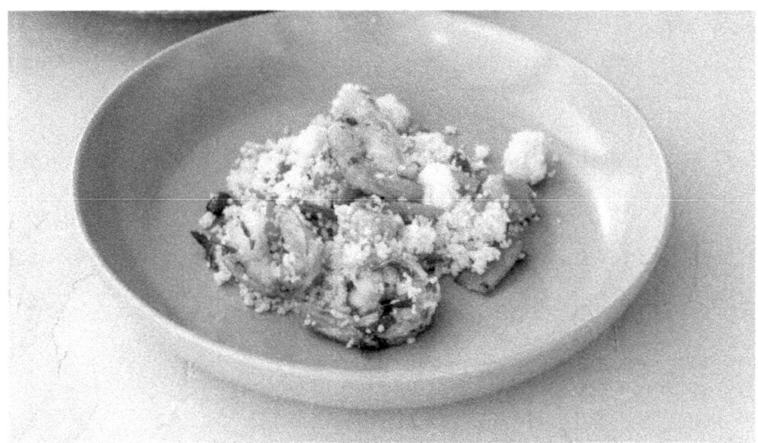

Cauliflower Fried Rice with Vegetables and Shrimp is a low-carb and healthy alternative to traditional fried rice. It is made by pulsing cauliflower in your food processor to create a rice-like texture and then stir-frying it with vegetables, such as carrot, pea and onion, and shrimp. It is a great source of protein, fiber and nutrients, making it a satisfying and nutritious meal. The dish can be customized with your favorite toppings and add-ins for a flavorful and healthy meal.

Prep Time / Cooking Time: 55 Minutes

Serving Size: 2 Persons

Ingredient List

1 cauliflower head

- 1/2 pound peeled and deveined shrimp
- 1/2 cup frozen peas
- 1/2 cup diced carrot
- 1/2 cup diced onion
- 2 minced garlic cloves
- 2 tablespoons vegetable oil
- 2 tablespoons soy sauce
- 1 teaspoon sesame oil
- 1/4 teaspoon black pepper
- 2 beaten eggs

XXXXXXXXXXXXXXXXX

Instructions

a) Cut the cauliflower into small florets and pulse it in the food processor until it resembles rice. Set aside.

b) In a large skillet, heat the vegetable oil over medium-high heat. Add the shrimp, then cook until pink, about 2-3 minutes per side. Remove from the skillet and set aside.

c) In the same skillet, add the peas, carrot, onion and garlic. Cook until tender, about 5-7 minutes.

d) Add the cauliflower to the skillet and stir to combine it with the vegetables. Cook for 5-7 minutes, stirring occasionally.

e) Push the cauliflower to one side of the skillet and add the eggs to the other side. Scramble the eggs until cooked through, about 2-3 minutes.

f) Add the shrimp back to the skillet, then stir to combine.

g) In a small bowl, whisk together the soy sauce, sesame oil and black pepper. Pour the sauce over the mixture and stir to combine.

h) Serve hot and enjoy!

My Words

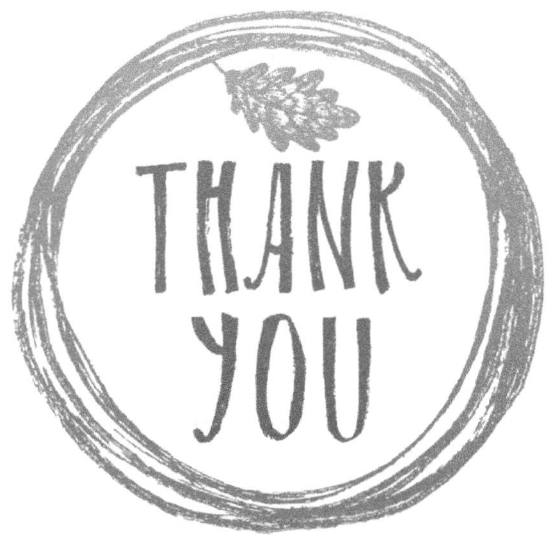

I cannot express enough how grateful I am for your decision to purchase my book. It is a humbling feeling to know that people are interested in learning from my experiences and the content that I have created. Being a writer has allowed me to share my knowledge and skills with others, and it is truly an honor to have you choose my book out of the multitude of books available on the market.

Your choice to invest in my book is incredibly special to me, and I am confident that the content you will find within its pages will prove to be valuable and insightful. It is my sincere hope that you will learn a great deal from the knowledge I have shared and that it will positively impact your life in some way.

After reading the book, I kindly request that you leave feedback, no matter how small. As a writer, I am always looking to improve and provide better content to my readers. Your feedback will be an invaluable source of information, and I will take it into consideration when creating future books. It is my goal to create content that my readers love and find helpful, and your input will play an important role in helping me achieve that.

Once again, I would like to express my gratitude for your support and for choosing my book. Your investment in my work means the world to me, and I am honored to have the opportunity to share my knowledge with you. Your feedback and support will be greatly appreciated and will help me to continue creating meaningful and valuable content for readers like you.

Kind regards,

Alex Aton